GRACE ATEA AMPOFOH

LIVING WITH DIABETES

— Metabolic Syndrome —

SECOND EDITION

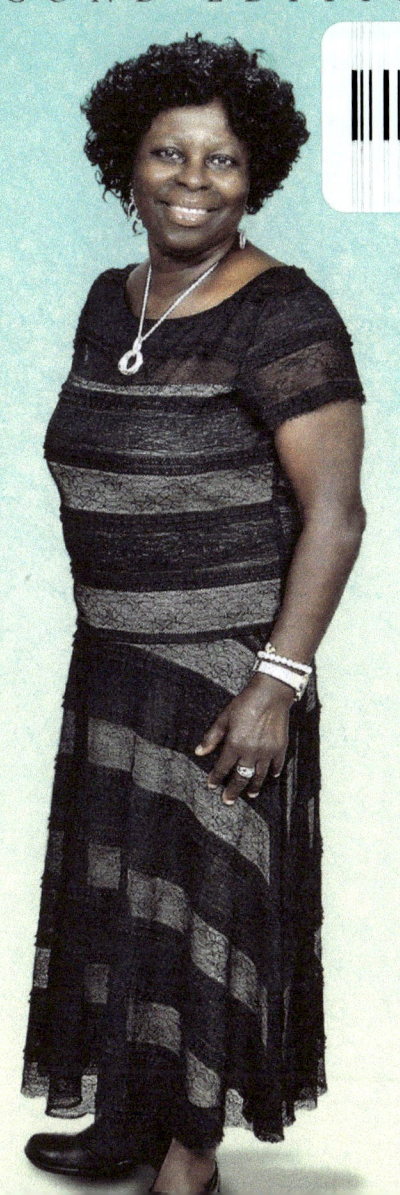

LIVING WITH
DIABETES
―― Metabolic Syndrome ――

LIVING WITH
DIABETES

—— Metabolic Syndrome ——

GRACE ATEA AMPOFOH

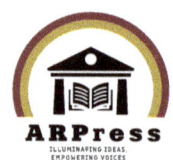

Copyright © 2021 by Grace Atea Ampofoh.

All rights reserved. No part of this publication may be reproduced, distributed, or transmitted in any form or by any means, including photocopying, recording, or other electronic or mechanical methods, without the prior written permission of the copyright owner and the publisher, except in the case of brief quotations embodied in critical reviews and certain other noncommercial uses permitted by copyright law. For permission requests, write to the publisher, addressed "Attention: Permissions Coordinator," at the address below.

ARPress
45 Dan Road Suite 5
Canton MA 02021

Hotline: 1(800) 220-7660
Fax: 1(855) 752-6001

Ordering Information:
Quantity sales. Special discounts are available on quantity purchases by corporations, associations, and others. For details, contact the publisher at the address above.

Printed in the United States of America.

 ISBN-13:   Paperback   979-8-89389-745-6
             eBook   979-8-89389-746-3

Library of Congress Control Number: 2021909692

Contents

Dedication vi

Aknowledgement vii

Chapter 1   Introduction 1

Chapter 2   What is Diabetes? 3

Chapter 3   Digestion Process 5

Chapter 4   Metabolic Syndrome 6

Chapter 5   Types of Diabetes 8

Chapter 6   Diabetes Myths and Misconceptions 13

Chapter 7   Somogyi Effect, Dawn Phenomenon 16

Chapter 8   Self- Management for Diabetes is
Necessary at All Times 19

Chapter 9   Home Management Activities 22

References 25

Inspirational Page 26

Author's Biography 30

Dedication

DEDICATED:
To Diabetes Research and Awareness of
Diabetes Self- Management.

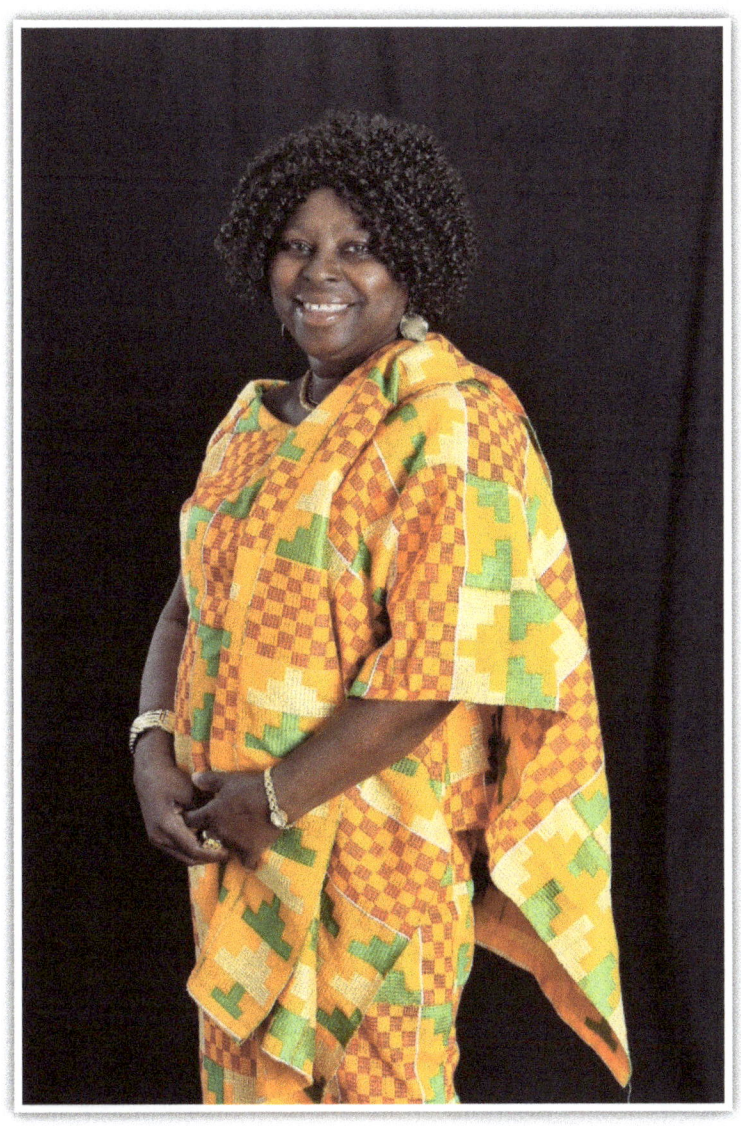

Aknowledgement

My sincere thanks go to the Publishers for assisting me to get the book published. I thank my friends and family for their support. I also owe a debt of gratitude to the experts who have dedicated their time sharing with us their various research works and opinions, and to promote how diabetes can be properly managed so at the end of the day, diabetics can live a healthy lifestyle. Lastly, I thank God for his grace.

CHAPTER 1

Introduction

At the age of 68, I am still determined to share my story with my audience, not as a motivational speaker, at least not for now, due to the outbreak of coronavirus-19 pandemic era, and the public health crisis. Why this era? My abrupt car accident in August, 2015 contributed to my physical disabilities. I was hit by a truck driver on my way home from the fitness center, after my routine exercises. My blood sugar was very low. I had no snack with me at that time. I had spinal stenosis, chronic back pain, migraine headaches, living with diabetes. The health care team did their best, but nothing helped me. I had surgery on the 28th of February, 2020. God has been good to me through it all. The beginning of my routine exercises after surgery and living with diabetes was not easy, especially after my spinal surgery. I walk for one hour or more a day now. I have faith in God to carry me through the storm.

Not too long ago, I watched a C-SPAN USA program on the television. It was a forum of panel debate on "Diabetes Research Report". Dear reader, I am determined wholeheartedly to share with you and all diabetics and their caretakers what I learned from this forum. This forum was educational, and as a student, I took some notes. Today, kidney transplant research has successfully been done to improve kidney disease treatment. Advance in technology has increased, and complication of diabetes has declined. New treatment by using autoimmune factor and stem cell to initiate treatment seems to work faster. Children diagnosed with Type-1 diabetes were among the participants. So one participant who was diagnosed with Type-1 diabetes at age 8, has improved due to advancement of treatment modalities. Now 17 years old, she is even an active musician. Another participant who was diagnosed with Type-1 diabetes was just 3 years old. Now, he has improved and grown as a successful student. He plays tennis, and enjoys golf and water sports. Some of the speakers were members of the US Senate. One member who also serve in the "Special Aging Committee", encouraged us to focus on the need to reduce the cost of INSULIN. He added that a NEW SPECIAL DIABETES PROGRAM is signed into law in in the US senate. Another speaker said, "ARTIFICIAL PANCREAS TREATMENT is used in my State in Nevada- U.S.A". One positive thing that challenged me was the report shared by Dr. Griffin Rogers, the director of "National Institute of Diabetes and Digestive and Kidney Disease". His remark was that, Kidney Transplant Treatment Research Work is being done. Dear reader, there is hope for better future, but some of the barriers of health care is " lack of education to the public in general regarding doses of insulin", he added.

CHAPTER 2

What is Diabetes?

Many experts have done numerous studies, including {CDC} Centers for Disease Control and Prevention report in the year 2020 on National diabetes statistics report, to define diabetes as a chronic {long lasting} disease that affects how your body turns or break down most of the food you eat into sugar {also called glucose} and release into your bloodstream. When your blood sugar goes up, it signals your pancreas to release insulin. Insulin acts like a key to let the blood sugar into your body cells for use as fuel or energy. Diabetes is a disorder of metabolism, thus the way our bodies use digested food for energy is abnormal. The disease involves several organs of the body and attacks different people in different ways. The exact cause is unknown. Dear reader, let me explain this concept once again. The answer is that diabetes is a disease in which the body does not produce or cannot properly use INSULIN, a hormone made by the pancreas.

The body uses insulin to convert sugar into the energy that powers us. Diabetes can also be described as a disease that makes it difficult for the body to turn food for energy. To understand DIABETES, it will be helpful to know about digestion process, metabolic syndrome, the function of the pancreas and insulin, and how all these relate to diabetes. We get sugar from two sources: In scenario 1, glucose is converted from the food we eat from starches and carbohydrates. In scenario 2, glucose is also manufactured in the liver and muscle. Diabetes is a condition that you must just live with longer and take good care of managing your disease, and your health in general. Although this might be hard, time consuming, and requires the help of tour loved ones, and good medical supervision. I strongly believe that diabetes must not slowly get worse or control your life. If you have diabetes, you have to work hard to achieve and maintain a healthy lifestyle. You can control prediabetes from slowly reaching Type-2 diabetes, and Type-2 from getting to complications of diabetes, including heart disease, stroke, nerve damage, eye disease, and kidney disease.

CHAPTER 3

Digestion Process

The mouth starts the process of food intake. The mouth chews and breaks up the food so it may be passed down to the stomach. Stomach and the intestines break down the food into nutrients and simpler substances the body can absorb. One of them is SIMPLE SUGAR or GLUCOSE. The pancreas produces hormones and substances that help with digestion. One of these hormones is INSULIN. The pancreas releases insulin into your blood circulation which help glucose to enter various cells in the body and be stored. The problem arises if your body does not make enough insulin, or if the insulin does not work the way it should, glucose in this case, cannot get into the body cells. But it stays in your blood, causing your blood glucose level to rise too high. Insulin is the key that allows glucose to enter into the cells. Let me compare glucose in your body, and gasoline in your car: Each is a fuel and a source of energy. If you run out of gasoline in your car, however, it is not enough to make the car move. You also need a key to start the motor, which allows the gasoline to be converted into energy. Like the car, your bodies also need a key that enables you to use glucose as energy. INSULIN is the key: It opens the door to allow GLUCOSE to pass from the bloodstream into the cells, where it produces energy for the body.

CHAPTER 4

Metabolic Syndrome

What is metabolic syndrome? Some experts describe this as a pattern, insulin- resistance syndrome. It is a collection of conditions that when taken together increases the risk of heart disease, stroke, and diabetes. Metabolic syndrome is the main deviation from the normal digestive function in the body system. A diagnosis of metabolic syndrome is made if a person has any three of the following risk factors: ABDOMINAL OBESITY or LARGE WAIST CIRCUMFERENCE, at least greater than forty {40} inches in men and greater than thirty-five {35} inches in women; fasting blood glucose at least 100mg/Dl; serum triglycerides at least 150mg/Dl; blood pressure {B/P} at least 135/85mmHg; HDL {"good"} cholesterol lower than 40 mg/Dl for men or 50mg/Dl for women. World Health Organization {WHO} emphasizes more on high glucose levels, impaired glucose tolerance test, and fasting glucose as they indicate that the person has diabetes; insulin resistance and protein in urine; urinary albumin secretion rate of 20mg/ minute or higher; and albumin to creatinine ratio/ GFR {30mg/minute or higher} are a/so positive factors. Active attention must be given to the need of prevention, and treatment to restore healthy lifestyle. Serious complications always arise in the negative way. Metabolic syndrome appears to affect between 25-30 percent {%} of the United States population, according to various national surveys. In fact, the number of people with metabolic syndrome seems to increase as we get older in our seventies {70}.

Symptoms and Causes

Usually there are no immediate physical symptoms. People with metabolic syndrome do have a tendency to be overweight, especially, around the abdomen, like an apple shape. Since the condition is associated with insulin resistance, the individuals with this condition may display some of the clinical symptoms of an increase in the production of insulin. For example, women may experience cysts in their ovaries or irregular menstrual periods, conditions associated with metabolic syndrome. Consistently, high levels of insulin are associated with many harmful diseases in the body before its manifestation as a disease. The cause is unknown. According to experts' opinion, it is influenced in most cases by DIET and LIFESTYLE. It is also genetically driven. Many features of metabolic syndrome are associated with insulin resistance as well, but the negative result is that it causes the body cells to lose their sensitivity to insulin.

CHAPTER 5

Types of Diabetes

PREDIABETES: This is an early warning sign of metabolic syndrome that can lead to developing type-2 diabetes. The good news is that maintaining a healthy weight and being physically active can often reverse the condition and delay or prevent the development of type- 2 diabetes. You need to be under good medical supervision to screen you and rule out the warning signs and the risk factors for prediabetes which are as follows:

1. Are you overweight? Studies show that being overweight alone contributes more than fifty percent {50%} risk factor for developing diabetes, more so without physical activity. Obesity doubles sixteenth {16th} fold risk for diabetes compared to active person, while inactive lean person risks double to develop diabetes.

2. Do you have excess weight around your waist?

3. Is your diet high in Carbohydrates, such as white bread, potatoes and pasta?

4. Do you eat starchy snacks food or sweets?

5. Do you exercise less than three {3} hours per week?

6. Are you African- American, Hispanic –American, Native American, Asian-American or Pacific Islander? They have higher risk for developing diabetes.

7. Do you have family history of diabetes, including father, mother, or siblings.

8. Do you have high blood pressure over 140/90mm/hg?

9. Do you have high Cholesterol?

10. Are you over forty-five {45} years old?

High blood sugar levels over months and years in most cases can lead to serious complications. For most people, the higher the blood sugar level, the higher the chance of complications.

Extremely high blood sugar levels can cause loss of consciousness, and even death. Overall the risk of death is twice as high with people with diabetes than those without the disease. Therefore you should pay attention to screening and prevention of diabetes and its complications.

TYPE-1 DIABETES: For some people with diabetes, insulin is not able to carry out its function for one of two reasons: The pancreas may not produce enough insulin. In some cases your pancreas is no longer producing insulin, and this is why type-1 in also called "Insulin dependent diabetes mellitus {IDDM} ". In this case, the specialized beta cells of the pancreas stop producing insulin. The condition usually starts in childhood, and the people who are diagnosed with this condition require lifelong insulin therapy and careful dietary management to survive. Today, due to new medical interventions, STEM- CELL transplants have been used successfully in the treatment of type-1 diabetes. Most type-1 cases are caused by autoimmune disease, in which case the body mistakenly attacks and destroys the beta cells in the pancreas. Type-1 diabetes strikes suddenly. You may appear fine one day, and be very sick just a few weeks or even days later.

TYPE-2 DIABETES: In general, when we talk about diabetes we are referring to type-2 diabetes. About 90-95% cases of diabetes have type-2 diabetes, a disease that is quite different from type-1. In a large majority of cases, the individual still makes insulin. In fact, the person may make large amounts of insulin, but the cells do not open to allow the insulin in. Your body cells, as a diabetic, respond slowly to its presence. This condition is also known as insulin resistance. Over time, the rising of blood glucose levels become abnormal. What we see here simply, explains how insulin tries to knock hard at the cell walls and asks them to allow the blood glucose to enter. But the cells do mot open. This is why your blood glucose or sugar level increases {hyperglycemia}. But to force blood glucose to enter the cells, the pancreas pours out more insulin causing you to become HYPOGLYCEMIC, leading to lots of damage to the body organs. As time goes on, the pancreas fails to produce enough insulin at such high levels, and that is why insulin therapy is required in order to control hyperglycemia.

GESTATIONAL DIABETES: About 40% of pregnant women, each year in the United States of America develop gestational diabetes. The risk factors are women over 25 years old who are obese with increased blood sugar levels, hypertension, family history of diabetes, and people from certain ethnic groups. The outcome of women with gestational diabetes may be an infant with increased birth weight which causes difficulty during labor and delivery, including possibility of caesarean section. Risks to infants include high concentration of glucose levels in their blood before birth to the first few days postpartum. Breathing problem is most likely to occur and may require oxygen therapy if born early. Baby may become overweight and develop diabetes later on in life, because of inheriting mother's metabolic tendencies. You must be proactive to control gestational diabetes and find a new lifestyle by paying particular attention to the following measures:

1. Diet plan suitable for all diabetics.

2. Sensible exercise during pregnancy.

3. Monitor blood sugar levels frequently, and know the signs for your lows and highs so you can treat those warning signs better.

Blood glucose levels usually return to normal after delivery. However, about 20- 50% chance of developing type-2 diabetes within the next few years is possible.

Overview of Type-1 and Type-2 Diabetes.

	Type-1	Type-2
Characteristics	Insulin dependent	May or may not need insulin and oral medication.
Age	Begins before age 20 but begins After age 40 or earlier.	Can occur in adults.
Insulin	Little or none produced, insulin May not be enough.	It cannot be used.
Onset	Sudden	Slow
Gender	Both males and females.	More females are Affected.
Heredity	Some tendency.	Strong tendency.
Weight	Majority are thin/weight loss.	Overweight.
Ketones	Ketones present in urine.	No ketones in urine.
Treatment	Insulin, diet, exercise.	Diet, exercise, Medication.

CHAPTER 6

Diabetes Myths and Misconceptions

There are several myths, cultural beliefs, poverty, and lack of knowledge that can contribute to fear and apprehension about living with diabetes, and the fact that the disease will shorten your life, considering all the complications it entails. These statements bothered me for years because of many factors. Unfortunately, your response to these myths may cripple you stay still until you take your last breath instead of getting some help. It is sometimes very difficult to help someone else when you yourself happen to be in the same boat. Dear reader, I don't know about you, but it happened to me in my early years living with diabetes, due to anger and lack of support leading to failure to control my chronic diabetes, complications of diabetes including stroke, kidney and eye problems. My nerve damage was caused by my automobile accident in August, 2015. Yes, I was in the same bout back then, but reliable information about awareness of self- management of diabetes is available now. I want to talk to my audience about some of the MYTHS and MISCONCEPTIONS in relation to diabetes, in Q&A style.

1. Can you Develop Diabetes by Eating Sugar?

   Many people get confused when they hear this, but I learned that eating too much sugar will not cause diabetes. A person with diabetes has to watch for the total number of CALORIES on their plate. Calorie is the unit of fuel or energy of food. If you eat excessive calories of any kind, causing you to gain weight and develop insulin resistance, you may end up with diabetes. American Diabetes Association recommends that a healthy diet may include up to fifteen percent {15%} of its caloric content from simple sugar.

2. Is Insulin the number one therapy for diabetes?

   Insulin therapy can be avoided. Some experts argue that there are many alternatives to having to inject yourself more often. Insulin is not addictive, and it is not given as a drug. It is used as a replacement therapy for the naturally occurring hormone insulin. In a safer side, sometimes it is used in pregnancy, in some cases of infection, heart attack, or major surgical procedures. People may need insulin temporarily to control their sugar levels. This does not mean that in those circumstances, you will be on insulin the rest of your life. Actually, early treatment of insulin therapy may prevent diabetes complications, such as kidney disease, heart disease, eye, and nerve damage. Control of blood pressure and cholesterol levels are positive outcomes of insulin therapy. On the negative side, insulin therapy can be time consuming and demanding of a person's attention than exercise, diet, medication, and managing diabetes itself.

3. Can women with diabetes have children, or should they not have children?

There are women who may be afraid to have children, because of misconception. People with diabetes can have children. For example, I am a living testimony. I have children. There are some risks involved, because women with poorly controlled diabetes at the time of conception may experience problems. Some women are diagnosed with gestational diabetes, which puts both mother and baby into complication during pregnancy, labor and delivery. Some women recover after delivery, but there is high risk for developing Type- 2 diabetes later on in life.

CHAPTER 7

Somogyi Effect, Dawn Phenomenon

Certain individuals experience profuse early morning night sweat, and may be due to inadequate nighttime insulin doses. It may also be due to counter- regulatory hormones in the early morning hours. I had this problem for a long period in my life living with diabetes, due to poor medical supervision, poor self- care management of uncontrolled diabetes, and stress.

All the credit goes to the pioneer who discovered the chain of events which leads to rebound morning hyperglycemia. In December, 2014, Somogyi effect was updated, with a new definition that explains this effect in simple terms. It is caused by "nighttime hypoglycemia, which leads to rebound hyperglycemia in the early morning hours. In other words, when your blood sugar or glucose level drops at night during your sleep as a diabetic, it happens that in the early morning hours hormones are released which trigger the liver to release glucose, that cause your blood glucose level to rise when you wake up in the morning. This happens as a result of having extra insulin in the body before bedtime. This problem occurs in Type-1 diabetes. Some of the risk factors are the following: people on long acting insulin like Lantus, when you don't eat snack before bedtime, causing the blood sugar to drop early in the morning and the body to release hormones to counteract the drop. Another reason is that, it could be from the "dawn phenomenon" which happens during the night when hormones are released that trigger the liver to put out glucose. If there is not enough insulin in the body to counteract this then blood glucose level rise during the night, resulting in high glucose level in the morning. Both Somogyi effect, and dawn phenomenon are similar in a sense that they both lead high morning blood sugar levels as a result of hormones released that causes the liver also to release glucose into the bloodstream. The only difference is that dawn phenomenon is not caused by hyperglycemia, but just by the release of hormones. As glucose level in the blood increases, the pancreas tries to overcompensate and produce even more insulin which leads to the characteristic symptoms of metabolic syndrome. When insulin levels rise, a stress response occurs, that leads to elevations in the cortisol, the body's long - acting stress hormone. This, in turn, creates an inflammatory reaction that, if left untreated, begins to damage healthy tissue.

Some experts recommend that you eat light bedtime snack including some protein to keep glucose levels balanced with insulin. Check your blood sugar in the middle of the night if possible on several nights and around three o'clock in the morning. To determine if your blood- sugar is low. It is advisable for diabetics to keep and maintain medical supervision for their health care in general, and at all times, for successful outcome. In fact, it is possible to improve blood sugar level even if there is not very much reduction of the excess fat. Your journey back to health begins with improvement that will happen before losing all the weight. The weight loss may be slow or even nonexistence that is alright. Diet control is also an important aspect of diabetes self-management. Eat small, frequent meals, instead of large meals to that can flood the bloodstream with glucose and insulin. Diet control is an important issue in managing metabolic syndrome. Watch your portion of calorie on your plat. Keep fats and trans fats to minimum but take moderate amounts of non -saturated oil like, olive oil, some nuts, sardines, and Omega-3 oil. Eat more fish like wild cold water fish that are high in Omega-3 fatty acids, such as salmons and sardines. You can even take Omega-3 supplements. Eat more non- starchy vegetables like leafy green salad, cucumbers, bell peppers, eggplant, spinach, cabbage, mushroom, and broccoli.

CHAPTER 8

Self-Management for Diabetes is Necessary at All Times

LAB WORKS: Complete Blood Count/CBC

This test shows the state of your blood cells. Many people with diabetes develop anemia, meaning they have fewer red blood cells than they should. If your CBC is low, more investigations need to be done by your health care provider. Some of the causes of anemia may include kidney disease, iron deficiency anemia, and abnormal bleeding.

URINE TESTING/Fast fact

The first glucose monitor was invented in India years ago. A physician will spill sample of a patient's urine unto the ground, then study how fast ants would crawl towards the urine spot. Thus how the physician would be able to judge how high the patient's sugars were, in the urine. Urine tests for presence of sugar are still reliable methods used to check for KETONES in urine. When insulin levels are extremely low in people with type-1 diabetes, the body turns to fat for sources of energy and produces ketones, indicating that the individual's blood sugar levels are extremely high leading to ketoacidosis. Physicians may order frequent urine tests for ketones if their patients' sugar levels are running above 250-300mg/Dl. Today, some blood glucose monitors also can be used to check for KETONES in the blood routinely. Doctors also order tests for protein in urine routinely. If your urine tests positive for significant amount of albumin, then you should control your diabetes and blood pressure, and you may need special medications to protect your kidneys. When the kidneys filter the blood, excess glucose spills out in the urine, leading to secondary signs and symptoms of diabetes, such as frequent urination, and large amount of sugar in the urine, This is how diabetes got its name officially as DIABETES MELLITUS: Greek word diabetes = "to pass through" ; Latin word mellitus = "sugar/ honey". The good news is that plenty can be done to slow kidney damage.

HEMOGLOBIN A1C

This blood sugar test helps you and your doctor understand how well your treatment plan is working. This test shows your blood sugar levels over the last three {3} months. For many people with diabetes, A1C of less than 7% is a good goal. If your test result in every three months is over 7%, your doctor needs to change your treatment plan including diet to help control your high blood sugar levels, and your health in general. Each person has unique needs and goals and the doctor needs to plan for each diabetic patient as such for positive outcome.

FASTING PLASMA GLUCOSE {FPG} or CASUAL PLASMA GLUCOSE TEST.

According to Centers for Disease Control and Prevention {CDC}, millions of Americans are unaware that they have diabetes, because they may be no warning signs. To confirm diagnosis of type-2 diabetes, your doctor will order FPG or Casual Plasma Glucose test. This is a preferred method for diagnosing diabetes because it is easy to do, convenient and less expensive than other tests, according to American Diabetes Association {ADA}. Patient should fast at least eight hours prior to the test. Venous blood is drawn and sent to the laboratory for analysis. The result of 70- 100mg/Dl is normal for nondiabetics. When your readings for two separate fasting blood glucose levels are greater than or equal to 126mg/Dl, it indicates you are a diabetic.

GLUCOSE TOLERANCE TEST {GTT}

If your FPG is normal but you show some signs of risk factors, your doctor may order this test. The reasons are that blood sugar rises rapidly as you eat, or impaired glucose tolerance. If your blood sugar levels are high enough they may be diagnosed with diabetes. It is a time consuming and expensive test, but it is the best way the body reacts to carbohydrate intake. It is like making a movie of your metabolism. Experts have been able to research with data, comparing how insulin and blood sugar levels work as we consume carbohydrates. People with high risks for developing metabolic syndrome were easily identified. Proper education and intervention are necessary steps we can use to manage people with metabolic syndrome in order to prevent the development, or stop the progression of prediabetes and type-2 diabetes.

CHAPTER 9

Home Management Activities

It is important to wear a "diabetic bracelet" for emergency situations, or you can carry an emergency card in your wallet, including your doctor's phone number, medication lists and family contact information. Carry snack, candy or any remedy food, such as soda or fast – acting carbohydrate source with you to quickly manage a low blood sugar level. Dear reader, I want to share my personal testimony with you today for education. I worked as a night nurse for years before retirement, and what I used to do is to walk in the mornings around familiar neighborhood, for my routine exercises. Bad thing happened to me one day when I forgot to carry snack with me, just because I was rushing on that particular morning to fulfil my goal. My blood sugar dropped on my way home and I felt it. The situation was bad since there was no bracelet or contact information with me. Suddenly, I became confused, anxious to walk about one mile distance to go home. I didn't have my cell- phone on me. God was my witness, why I put myself in that plight for the need of exercising to lose weight in order to control diabetes. It was my best exercise in the journey so far. With poor gait, I tried to move to the sidewalk, and I was soaked and wet as sweat came down on my body like rain upon the grass in the early morning. As I was wondering how I could go back home, I saw a lady in a van near me, and I said to her. "I am a diabetic and my sugar is low, but I forgot my snack at home". The driver was confused, and that was what I thought. She said, "I see you walk by my house every morning". She meant I wasn't a stranger to her. As soon as she opened her car door for me, I jumped in and said, "thank you! My house is not far from here". I did not ask her any question because I was uncomfortable. Living with diabetes is not easy, especially if you have other underlying health problems such hypertension, high cholesterol, physical disability, stroke, eye problems, social isolation, etc. But one thing I know is that God is merciful. He sent his guardian angel to send me home. The lady was on her to work that morning, but she saw me at the right place, right time and did the right thing for sending me home in three minutes. May God bless her. I have not seen her since that day because I don't know her name or residence.

Questions/tips to ask yourself as a diabetic:

1. When you check your finger-stick for blood glucose level, was the result within the recommended range?

2. Are any of your numbers under or over your recommended target?

3. Do you notice any daily pattern?

4. Are there times during the day that your glucose is lower than target range?

5. Are there any specific times during the day that your glucose is higher than target range?

6. Can you think of any reason why your blood glucose acted as it did?

SAMPLE OF DAILY BLOOD GLUCOSE PROFILE.

Day 1: *5/16/2021*
When tested: *Before breakfast.*
Time of day: *7:00 am*
Blood glucose test results {mg/dL}: *120mg/dL*

If you have been managing your diabetes well, eating well, exercising and taking your medication, and your morning sugar result is still high------ you may be going to bed with your blood sugar within the target range, but your levels are high in the morning-------please refer to dawn phenomenon theory. To correct this, your doctor may base on the results of your blood testing results throughout the night or recommend you not to eat carbohydrates close to bedtime. Adjusting your dose of medication or insulin or switching to a different medication are other options of intervention

References

Vafcarie, L, LLC. Fat Belly Diet and Diabetes.

The American Association of Kidney Beginnings; Genetic Alliance Reprinted 2015, {www.aakp.org} Tampa FL-USA.

New York Times. "Learn to maintain a healthy lifestyle". New York –USA.

"Reverse Diabetes Forever" by Reader's Digest Association, INC, New York- USA

Frederic J. Vaguim MD, FACS & LD Chilnick, "The weight loss plan for beating diabetes"2009, Kaplan -New York.

Liz Vacceriello & Gillian Avarthuzik, RD. CDE, & Steven V. Edelman, MD, "Flat belly diet and diabetes", 2011, Dodale, New York- USA.

C- SPAN program – USA, July, 2019, "-Diabetes research report" –update.

Kenneth N. Anderson, & Lois E. Anderson, "Mosby's pocket dictionary of medicine, nursing, & allied health", 1990, the C. V. Mosby company, St Louis, MI- USA.

Inspirational Page

a. Lisa Torbert a yoga instructor said, "People are looking for ways to motivate their minds, bodies and spirits to get healthy". If your question is whether you can lose weight with yoga, her answer is yes! An hour of yoga can burn 250 calories. Yoga stretches muscles lengthwise, causing fat to be eliminated around the cells. She also said that a healthy diet is the foundation for a healthy lifestyle.

b. Nerve Damage: People with diabetes are at risk of nerve damage which can take two forms. Peripheral Neuropathy or Sensorimotor Neuropathy, which indicates the damage to the nerves that allows you to feel things or move your muscles. It leads to tingling sensation, pain, numbness or weakness in your feet or hands.

c. Autonomic Neuropathy: This is abnormality in the nerves that control your internal functions. It can lead to digestive problems, such as nausea, vomiting, constipation, or diarrhea. It can cause problems in the bladder control, or sexual function. Other symptoms include dizziness, fainting episodes, increased or decreased sweating, and visual problems adjusting to light and dark conditions. There may be lack of awareness if there is a warning sign of hypoglycemia. The key to prevention and treatment of neuropathy is to control your diabetes.

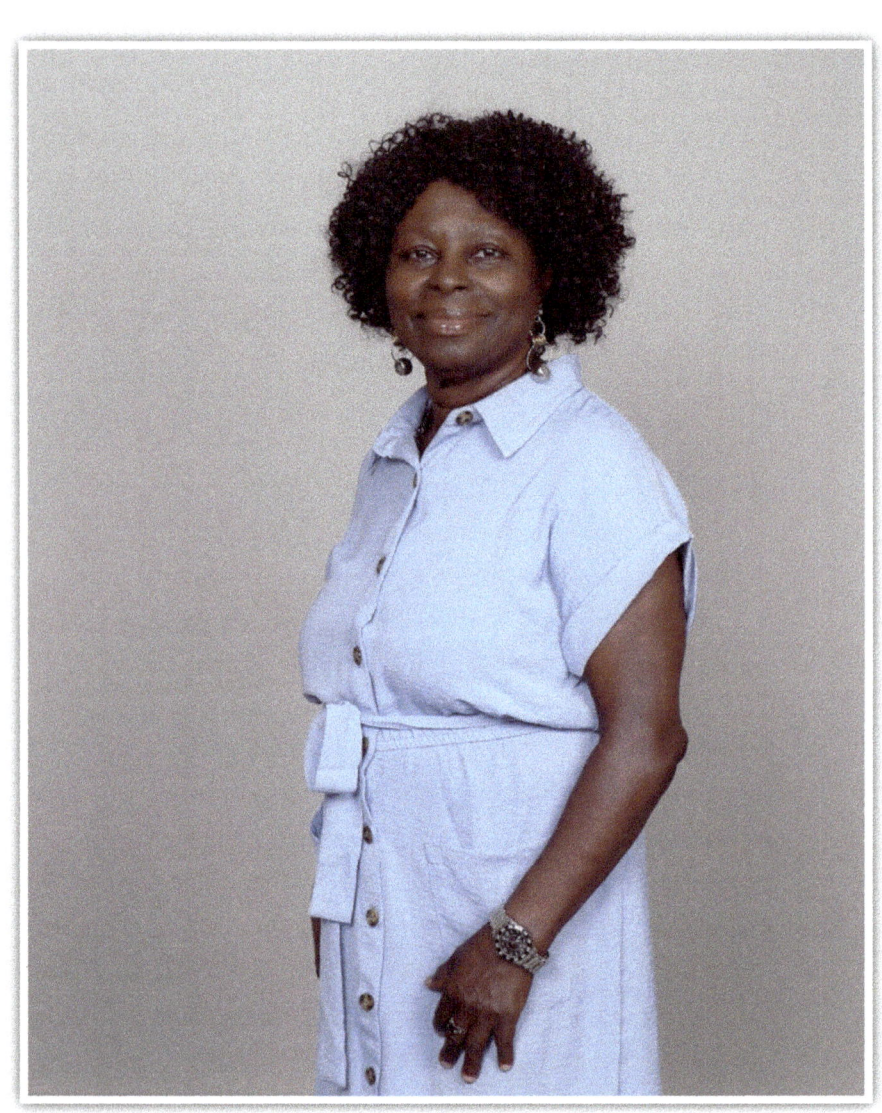

The book of PSALMS: This is a poetic book which forms another of the Bible's wonderful books. Psalms is a manual for devotional reading, and it can be read no matter what the condition of the reader's mind is or what his or her needs are. Every form of sorrow, joy, repentance, aspiration, prayer or hope finds expression in one or another of the psalms, such as follows:

Psalm. 1:1-2
1. Blessed is the man that walked not in the counsel of ungodly, nor standeth in the way of sinners, nor sitteth in the seat of the scornful.

2. But his delight is in the law of the LORD; and in his law doth he meditate day and night. Josh.1:8.

Psalm.100: 1-5.

A psalm of praise.
1. Make a joyful noise unto the LORD, all ye lands,

2. Serve the LORD with gladness; come before his presence with singing,

3. Know ye that the LORD he is God: it is he that hath made us, and not we ourselves; we are his people, and the sheep of his pasture.

4. Enter into his gate with thanksgiving, and into his courts with praise; be thankful unto him, and bless his name.

5. For the LORD is good; his mercy is everlasting; and his truth endureth to all generations.

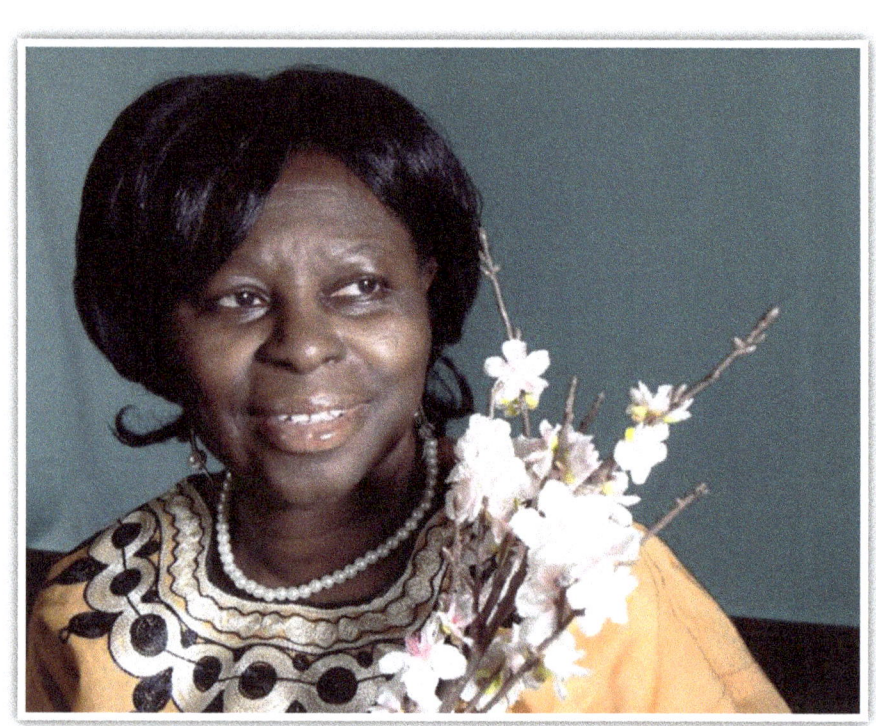

Author's Biography

Grace Atea Ampofoh is a sixty-eight-year old retired nurse in Delaware, United States of America who wants to share her story of life experiences living with diabetes, for empowerment. She is a strong believer in God, with a diploma in applied spirituality from the Christian Leadership University school of the spirit, Cheektowaga, New York. She has two successful daughters, and two granddaughters.

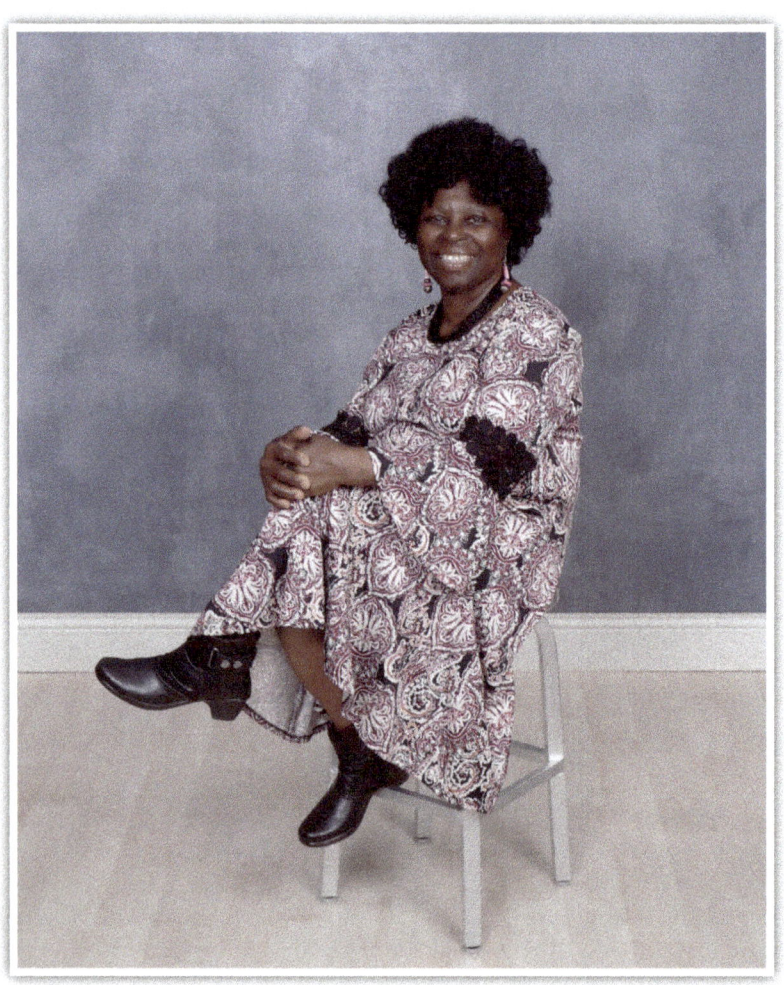